CHRONIC BRONCHITIS NUTRITION FOR BEGINNERS

Optimize Your Health With Targeted Dietary Approaches, Recipe Collections, And Proven Lifestyle Adjustments For Chronic Bronchitis Relief

DR. JACE ZAYDEN

Table of Contents

DISCLAIMER

The information provided in the book is intended for general informational purposes only. The content of this book should not be considered a substitute for professional medical advice, diagnosis, or treatment.

Readers are advised to consult with a qualified healthcare professional for medical advice tailored to their individual circumstances.

The author has made every effort to ensure that the information in this book is accurate and up-to-date at the time of publication. However, medical knowledge is constantly evolving, and new research may emerge that could impact the information presented. The author disclaims any responsibility for any adverse effects or consequences resulting from the use of the information provided in this book.

References or mentions of individuals, products, websites, organizations, or other names within this book are for informational purposes only and do not constitute an endorsement. The author has no affiliations with, and makes no endorsements of, any third-party entities mentioned. Readers are encouraged to conduct their own research and exercise their judgment when considering any external resources or recommendations.

The author and the publisher shall have neither liability nor responsibility to any person or entity with respect to any loss, damage, or injury caused or alleged to be caused directly or indirectly by the information contained in this book. Any reliance on the information within this book is at the reader's own risk.

By reading this book, the reader acknowledges and agrees to the terms of this disclaimer. If the reader does not agree with these terms, they should not use the information provided in this book.

ABOUT THIS BOOK

"Chronic Bronchitis Nutrition" is an all-encompassing manual that explores the complex correlation between nutrition and chronic bronchitis management. This book commences with a perceptive preface that establishes the context for comprehending the importance of nutrition in the context of managing chronic bronchitis. In the following section, titled "Understanding Chronic Bronchitis," a comprehensive outline of the condition is presented, establishing the groundwork for the pivotal significance of nutrition in its successful control.

The central argument of this book is to underscore the criticality of nutrition in the context of chronic bronchitis management. This statement emphasizes the critical significance of dietary decisions in mitigating symptoms and improving the overall well-being of individuals afflicted with this respiratory ailment.

The "Dietary Guidelines for Chronic Bronchitis Patients" chapter functions as a pragmatic guide, providing explicit and implementable recommendations for individuals who are confronted with the task of regulating their condition through dietary choices.

Critical to this book's argument is its examination of vital nutrients that are indispensable for respiratory health. The chapter titled "Key Nutrients for Respiratory Health" offers a comprehensive analysis of the essential nutrients that are critical for the preservation of peak lung function and the mitigation of chronic bronchitis symptoms. Additionally, it offers pragmatic recommendations for integrating these nutrients into one's daily dietary regimen.

This book not only imparts theoretical understanding but also furnishes practical instruments for the execution of dietary modifications. This book outlines "Foods to Include in a Chronic Bronchitis Diet" and "Foods to Avoid in Chronic Bronchitis" provide precise suggestions supported by scientific evidence, aiming to enable individuals to make well-informed decisions concerning their dietary consumption. Acknowledging the importance of hydration, this book delves into the function of water in the context of chronic bronchitis, offering valuable perspectives on the maintenance of proper fluid equilibrium.

An additional emphasis is placed on practicality in the book "Meal Planning for Chronic Bronchitis Patients," which provides a methodical framework for individuals to integrate nutritious eating practices into their everyday schedules. The recognition that "Nutritional Supplements for Chronic Bronchitis" is incorporated into the list signifies that supplements may have the capacity to improve respiratory health.

In addition to discussing dietary changes, this book also explores lifestyle adjustments that may potentially enhance respiratory well-being. Chapters such as "Special Considerations for Chronic Bronchitis and Coexisting Conditions" and "Monitoring and Managing Weight in Chronic Bronchitis" offer a comprehensive perspective on the management of chronic bronchitis.

Acknowledging the collaborative nature of the healthcare sector, this book concludes by providing recommendations on "Collaborating with Dietitians and Healthcare Professionals," underscoring the criticality of employing a multidisciplinary methodology to ensure comprehensive care. "Chronic Bronchitis Nutrition" is an exceptional resource that provides a comprehensive combination of scientific insights and pragmatic guidance to enable individuals to proactively manage their nutritional decisions and, by extension, enhance their respiratory well-being.

CHAPTER ONE

Introduction

Prolonged inflammation of the bronchial tubes is known as chronic bronchitis, which is distinguished by the presence of coughing, mucous production, and respiratory distress. The development of this respiratory ailment is frequently correlated with prolonged exposure to irritants, including air pollution and cigarette smoke. Although medical intervention is of utmost importance in the management of chronic bronchitis, it is equally vital to recognize the significant impact that nutrition has on promoting general health and mitigating symptoms.

This book examines the foundational aspects of chronic bronchitis, emphasizes the critical role that nutrition plays in its management, and offers dietary recommendations to improve the overall health of those who are afflicted with this condition.

Comprehension Of Chronic Bronchitis

Chronic bronchitis, which causes increased mucous production, is a form of chronic obstructive pulmonary disease (COPD) characterized by inflammation and constriction of the bronchial passages. Prolonged exposure to irritants that induce airway injury is the principal etiology. Persistent cough, excessive mucous production, dyspnea, and chest pain are typical symptoms. As chronic bronchitis progresses, it can have a substantial detrimental effect on an individual's quality of life; therefore, it is critical to implement a holistic approach to its control.

In conjunction with pharmaceutical interventions like bronchodilators and anti-inflammatory drugs, lifestyle adjustments, encompassing appropriate nutrition, are integral facets of the management of chronic bronchitis. The function of nutrition in immune system support, inflammation reduction, and overall respiratory health optimization is crucial. Potential benefits of dietary modification for individuals with chronic bronchitis include symptom relief and an overall improvement in health.

The Significance Of Nutrition In The Management Of Chronic Bronchitis

Consistent nutrition is critical for individuals afflicted with chronic bronchitis due to the numerous positive effects it can have on their overall well-being. An optimally balanced diet has the potential to enhance respiratory function, decrease inflammation, and bolster the immune system. Additionally, proper nutrition can contribute to weight maintenance, which is critical for those with chronic bronchitis because obesity can place excessive pressure on the respiratory system.

Specific nutrients have been recognized for their potential therapeutic advantages in the management of chronic bronchitis. Vitamins C and E, among other antioxidants, can aid in preventing oxidative stress and inflammation in the airways. Salmon, flaxseeds, and walnuts contain omega-3 fatty acids, which possess anti-inflammatory properties that could prove advantageous for those afflicted with chronic bronchitis. Furthermore, it is critical to ensure adequate vitamin D levels for optimal respiratory health, as it has been associated with a decreased likelihood of developing respiratory infections.

Protein consumption is essential for those afflicted with chronic bronchitis, as it aids in the repair and preservation of tissues, including those comprising the respiratory muscles. Incorporate protein-dense foods into one's diet, including lean meats, poultry, fish, lentils, and legumes, to promote optimal respiratory function.

Dietary Guidelines For Patients With Chronic Bronchitis

1. Placing Great Emphasis on Fruits and Vegetables: An intake abundant in fruits and vegetables satisfies the need for antioxidants, vitamins, and minerals. These nutrients aid in the reduction of airway inflammation and promote overall health. Aim to consume an assortment of

vibrant fruits and vegetables to obtain a wide variety of nutrients.

2. Omega-3 Fatty Acids: Incorporate omega-3 fatty acid sources, such as flaxseeds, chia seeds, pecans, and rich fish (salmon, mackerel), into your diet. The anti-inflammatory properties of these lipids may aid in the relief of chronic bronchitis symptoms.

3. To ensure optimal vitamin D levels, allocate time for outdoor activities that facilitate the body's natural production of vitamin D via solar exposure. Furthermore, incorporate vitamin D-rich foods, such as fortified dairy products, fatty salmon, and egg yolks, into your dietary regimen.

4. Give precedence to lean protein sources: Incorporate lean protein sources into your dietary regimen to promote respiratory function and muscle health. Skinless poultry, lean portions of meat, fish, lentils, and legumes are all viable alternatives.

5. Maintaining adequate hydration is of the utmost importance for those who have chronic bronchitis. The thinned and more manageable mucus produced by water facilitates the clearing of the airways. Make it a priority to consume sufficient water throughout the day.

6. Restrict Intake of Processed Foods and Sugar: Tobacco products and foods that are loaded with added carbohydrates have the potential to exacerbate respiratory symptoms and promote inflammation. Consume only minimally processed, whole foods; limit your consumption of sugary munchies and beverages.

7. Maintain a healthy weight by adhering to a well-balanced dietary regimen and engaging in consistent physical activity. Chronic bronchitis patients may find it more difficult to breathe comfortably due to the respiratory distress caused by excess weight.

8. It is advisable for individuals with chronic bronchitis to adopt the practice of eating smaller,

more frequent meals as opposed to larger, heavier ones. This can effectively mitigate symptoms of fullness and discomfort, thereby facilitating easier respiration.

Adopting a nutrient-dense and nutritionally balanced diet is, in summary, an essential component in the management of chronic bronchitis. Nutrition is of paramount importance in promoting holistic well-being, mitigating the inflammatory response, and enhancing respiratory functionality. By adopting these dietary recommendations into their daily routines, those who have chronic bronchitis can proactively enhance their quality of life and improve their overall health.

Nutrition For Chronic Bronchitis: Supporting The Respiratory System

Chronic bronchitis is a respiratory ailment distinguished by inflammation of the bronchial passages, which results in chronic coughing, excessive secretion of mucous, and respiratory distress. Although medical intervention is of the utmost importance in the management of chronic bronchitis, adequate nutrition is equally critical in promoting respiratory health and mitigating symptoms. This article explores essential nutrients that are crucial for respiratory health, as well as recommendations for foods to incorporate into a diet for chronic bronchitis and those to exclude to encourage a holistic approach to managing this condition.

CHAPTER TWO

Essential Nutrients For Healthy Respiration

A harmonious equilibrium of vital nutrients is necessary for the preservation of respiratory health, as these nutrients support pulmonary function, the immune system, and general welfare. Several essential nutrients are pivotal in the management of chronic bronchitis:

1. This antioxidant vitamin is recognized for enhancing the immune system. It supports the immune system and aids in the fight against inflammation, both of which are crucial for those with chronic bronchitis. Bell peppers, citrus fruits, melons, and kiwis are all rich in vitamin C.

2. Vitamin D, which is frequently called the "sunshine vitamin," is critical for the regulation of the immune system. Supplements, fortified dairy products, fatty fish, and sunlight exposure can all aid in the maintenance of adequate vitamin D levels.

3. Omega-3 fatty acids, which are present in flaxseeds, salmon, and mackerel, are oily fish that contain anti-inflammatory properties. By including these in one's diet, inflammation in the respiratory tract can be reduced.

4. Zinc: This mineral is involved in wound healing and immune function. Zinc-rich foods, including legumes, lean proteins, nuts, and seeds, may promote respiratory health.

5. Antioxidants: Beta-carotene, selenium, and quercetin are among the numerous antioxidants that aid in the neutralization of free radicals and the reduction of inflammation.

Green tea, carrots, sweet potatoes, almonds, and seeds are all excellent sources of these antioxidants.

6. Sufficient protein consumption is essential for the preservation of respiratory muscle strength and optimal bodily operation. Legumes, lean meats, poultry, fish, and tofu are all superb sources of protein.

7. Maintaining adequate hydration is critical for the thinning of mucus and the enhancement of pulmonary function. Those who suffer from chronic bronchitis should strive to consume copious amounts of water daily.

Incorporating Foods Into A Diet For Chronic Bronchitis

A nutrient-dense, well-balanced diet can aid in the management of chronic bronchitis symptoms and enhance respiratory health as a whole. Incorporating the subsequent ingredients into a chronic bronchitis diet is advisable:

1. A diverse assortment of fruits and vegetables offers an extensive quantity of antioxidants, vitamins, and minerals. Cruciferous vegetables, verdant greens, berries, and citrus fruits have the potential to provide notable health benefits.

2. Omega-3 fatty acids, which are present in fatty fish such as salmon, trout, and mackerel, support respiratory function and have anti-inflammatory properties.

3. Nuts and Seeds: Rich in protein, antioxidants, and omega-3 fatty acids, almonds, walnuts, chia seeds, and flaxseeds all support respiratory health.

4. Consume lean proteins such as poultry, lean meats, tofu, and legumes to bolster the immune system and increase muscle strength.

5. Whole grains, including quinoa, brown rice, and whole wheat, are rich in fiber, complex carbohydrates, and vital nutrients.

6. Herbs and spices that possess anti-inflammatory properties and potentially ameliorate respiratory symptoms include ginger, turmeric, garlic, and oregano.

7. Incorporating hydrating foods into one's diet, such as watermelon, cucumber, and celery, can significantly enhance overall hydration.

Preventable Foods For Chronic Bronchitis

Certain foods have the potential to aggravate symptoms of chronic bronchitis by increasing inflammation and mucus production. Patients diagnosed with this condition may benefit from restricting or abstaining from the following:

1. Dairy products have the potential to induce increased mucus production in certain individuals. Dairy consumption should be reduced or eliminated if it exacerbates respiratory symptoms.

2. Processed food items, which contain elevated quantities of unhealthy lipids, sodium, and sugar, have the potential to impede respiratory health and exacerbate inflammation.

3. Caffeine and alcohol have the potential to cause dehydration in the body, which may result in mucous becoming thicker and airway clearance becoming more challenging.

4. Consuming an overabundance of sugary foods has the potential to worsen inflammation and undermine immune function. Restricting added carbohydrates improves health in general.

5. Fatty and seared foods have the potential to exacerbate inflammation and have adverse effects on respiratory function.

6. Spicy foods may elicit an exacerbation of wheezing and irritation of the airways in certain individuals. Consider your tolerance levels.

In summary, adherence to a meticulously designed chronic bronchitis diet, which prioritizes essential nutrients while avoiding potential triggers, can substantially aid in symptom management and the maintenance of respiratory health. It is of the utmost importance that people with chronic bronchitis collaborate with nutritionists and healthcare professionals to customize dietary recommendations to their particular requirements and preferences. The integration of a balanced and nourishing dietary regimen with medical treatment has the potential to significantly improve the general health and quality of life of individuals afflicted with chronic bronchitis.

The Importance Of Hydration In Chronic Bronchitis

The management of chronic bronchitis, which is distinguished by inflammation of the bronchial passages resulting in persistent coughing and respiratory difficulties, is significantly influenced by adequate hydration. It is critical for those with chronic bronchitis to maintain adequate hydration, as it aids in symptom relief and promotes overall respiratory health.

Sufficient hydration is critical for preserving the fluid and slender consistency of mucus produced in the respiratory system. Overproduction of mucus is a prevalent manifestation of chronic bronchitis, which results in respiratory distress and congestion. Adequate water consumption can aid in the prevention of mucous from solidifying and adhering, thereby facilitating its expulsion via wheezing.

In addition, proper hydration is crucial for averting dehydration, a condition that can worsen symptoms and impede the process of recovery. Mucus that is denser and more difficult to remove due to dehydration can exacerbate respiratory distress.

Individuals with chronic bronchitis should strive to consume a minimum of eight 8-ounce containers of water daily to maintain adequate hydration. Moreover, incorporating water-dense foods into one's diet, such as fruits and vegetables, can enhance overall hydration.

Although water is the most important fluid for sustaining proper hydration, individuals diagnosed with chronic bronchitis should restrict their consumption of alcoholic and caffeinated beverages. These substances have the potential to worsen respiratory symptoms and contribute to dehydration. Conversely, warm broths and herbal beverages offer additional hydration and provide solace without the adverse effects associated with caffeine and alcohol.

In conclusion, proper hydration is an essential component in the management of chronic bronchitis. It supports the body's natural defense mechanisms, aids in maintaining the thin consistency of mucous, and prevents dehydration, thereby contributing to overall respiratory health.

CHAPTER THREE

Meal Planning For Patients With Chronic Bronchitis

Adequate meal planning is of the utmost importance for those who suffer from chronic bronchitis, given that specific dietary decisions can either mitigate or worsen symptoms.

A nutritionally balanced diet has the potential to reduce inflammation, support the immune system, and supply the essential nutrients required for optimal respiratory health.

Including anti-inflammatory foods in meal planning for individuals with chronic bronchitis is a critical factor to consider. Fatty fish (salmon, mackerel, and trout), flaxseeds, and walnuts, which are abundant in omega-3 fatty acids, possess anti-inflammatory characteristics that may aid in the mitigation of inflammation within the bronchial passages. Moreover, antioxidant-rich fruits and vegetables, including verdant greens, citrus fruits, and berries, can provide support for the immune system.

Patients suffering from chronic bronchitis must incorporate lean protein sources into their diet. Protein is essential for the repair and maintenance of muscles, especially respiratory muscles. Included among the best sources of protein are poultry, lean meats, fish, tofu, and legumes.

Whole cereals, fruits, and vegetables ought to be the sources of carbohydrates to supply sustained energy and vital nutrients. Limit one's consumption of refined carbohydrates, which are present in white flour products and sweetened treats, due to their potential to exacerbate inflammation and adversely affect overall health.

In addition to the variety of foods ingested, the frequency of meals is also crucial. People with chronic bronchitis may benefit from smaller, more frequent meals as opposed to large, infrequent ones, to prevent the digestive system from becoming overloaded and the respiratory muscles from being overworked.

Maintaining a nutrient-dense and nutritionally balanced diet is fundamental in the management of chronic bronchitis. Seeking guidance from a registered dietitian or healthcare professional can assist in customizing a meal plan to suit specific needs and guarantee adherence to nutritional requirements.

Supplemental Diets For Chronic Bronchitis

In the management of chronic bronchitis, nutritional supplements may be of assistance by compensating for specific nutrient deficiencies and enhancing respiratory health as a whole. While obtaining the majority of nutrients from a balanced diet is essential, individuals with chronic bronchitis may benefit from certain supplements.

As a potent antioxidant, vitamin C provides immune system support. Vitamin C supplements may be beneficial for patients with chronic bronchitis, particularly when they experience heightened respiratory distress. Additionally, vitamin C-rich foods, including bell peppers, citrus fruits, and strawberries, may be incorporated into the diet.

Fish oil supplements contain omega-3 fatty acids, which have the potential to mitigate inflammation in the airways. In conjunction with dietary sources of omega-3s, these supplements may offer an extra anti-inflammatory benefit.

Potential immune system benefits of probiotics, which support a healthy balance of intestinal flora, are worthy of consideration. An association has been established between a balanced intestinal microbiome and general health; probiotic-rich foods or supplements may help maintain this equilibrium.

Specific minerals, including selenium and magnesium, are involved in antioxidant defense and muscle function. Foods that are abundant in magnesium include almonds, seeds, and leafy vegetables. On the other hand, selenium can be acquired from whole grains, seafood, and Brazil nuts. Supplementation may be required to address deficiencies in certain circumstances.

It is imperative to specify that the utilization of nutritional supplements ought to be conducted in the presence of a healthcare professional. Particular vitamins and minerals can cause adverse effects when consumed in excess, and individual requirements vary. A healthcare professional is capable of evaluating an individual's nutritional status and prescribing suitable supplements according to their particular needs.

Adjustments To One's Lifestyle To Enhance Respiratory Health

In addition to dietary adjustments, lifestyle modifications play a crucial role in the management of chronic bronchitis and the advancement of respiratory health. Individuals with chronic bronchitis can improve their overall quality of life by implementing healthier practices that enhance lung function and alleviate symptoms.

1. Cessation of smoking represents the most efficacious strategy for smokers to impede the advancement of chronic bronchitis. In addition to mitigating airway irritation, smoking cessation also reduces the likelihood of contracting respiratory infections.

2. Engaging in consistent physical activity can enhance respiratory function and contribute positively to the health of the lungs. Consistently participating in physical activity serves to fortify the respiratory muscles, improve cardiovascular health, and facilitate enhanced oxygen utilization. Engaging in activities such as yoga, walking, and swimming can yield notable advantages.

3. Avoiding Environmental Triggers: For the effective management of chronic bronchitis, it is vital to identify and avoid environmental triggers such as allergens, pollen, and air pollution. By employing air purifiers, donning masks when

required, and maintaining spotless living areas, one can reduce exposure to irritants.

4. Maintaining a Healthy Weight: Being overweight can place additional stress on the respiratory system, resulting in impaired respiration. By maintaining a healthy weight and achieving it through a balanced diet and regular exercise, the strain on the airways can be alleviated.

5. The management of chronic tension is crucial to safeguard respiratory health. The integration of stress-relieving practices, such as engaging in pastimes, meditation, or deep breathing exercises, can significantly enhance one's overall state of well-being.

6. Consistent Health Examinations: Consistent medical examinations are critical for monitoring respiratory function and promptly addressing any emergent concerns. Systematic evaluations enable medical practitioners to modify therapeutic strategies and administer essential interventions.

In summary, the effective management of chronic bronchitis requires a comprehensive strategy that integrates appropriate dietary practices, targeted dietary supplements, and wholesome lifestyle adjustments.

Under the supervision of healthcare professionals, individualized care can enable patients with chronic bronchitis to assume responsibility for their respiratory health and enhance their quality of life.

CHAPTER FOUR

Supporting The Respiratory System

Chronic bronchitis, which falls under the category of chronic obstructive pulmonary disease (COPD), is distinguished by ongoing inflammation of the airways, which results in a persistent cough and an accumulation of mucous. Although medical interventions are of utmost importance in the management of this condition, nutrition is equally critical in promoting respiratory health and overall wellness.

An essential component of nutrition for individuals with chronic bronchitis is the maintenance of a balanced diet. Sufficient nutrition is imperative for individuals afflicted with chronic bronchitis to bolster their respiratory function, fortify their immune system, and mitigate fatigue.

Consisting of a diet abundant in fruits, vegetables, whole cereals, and lean proteins enables one to replenish vital nutrients that fortify bodily systems and alleviate symptoms.

Nutritional recommendations for individuals with chronic bronchitis frequently prioritize foods rich in anti-inflammatory and antioxidant properties. Antioxidants, which are present in vegetables and fruits including berries, citrus fruits, spinach, and kale, reduce inflammation and combat oxidative stress. The incorporation of omega-3 fatty acids, which can be found in flaxseeds and fatty fish (salmon, mackerel), may additionally facilitate the anti-inflammatory response and conceivably alleviate symptoms.

Constant hydration is an essential requirement for those afflicted with chronic bronchitis. Adequate hydration facilitates the maintenance of mucous in a thin, manageable state, thereby enhancing the ease of airway clearance. For hydration, water, herbal beverages, and broths are all excellent options. Notwithstanding this, caffeine-containing beverages should be consumed with caution, as an overabundance of caffeine can result in dehydration.

In addition to the importance of a balanced diet, portion control is also vital. Weight gain can result from overeating, which can place additional stress on the respiratory system. Weight management and general health can be enhanced through the integration of regular, moderate physical activity into daily routines and the monitoring of caloric intake.

Weight Management And Monitoring In Patients With Chronic Bronchitis: Achieving Equilibrium

Effective weight management is an essential component of caring for individuals with chronic bronchitis, given that excessive weight can worsen respiratory symptoms and impair general health. On the contrary, being underweight may result in fatigue and muscle frailty. Achieving an optimal equilibrium is crucial in enhancing the quality of life for those afflicted with chronic bronchitis.

An inherent obstacle in the realm of weight management for individuals diagnosed with chronic bronchitis pertains to the condition's prospective influence on energy expenditure. Enhanced respiratory exertion may result in an increased expenditure of calories, thereby presenting difficulties for individuals in their pursuit of weight maintenance or gain. This underscores the importance of a meticulously customized nutrition regimen that addresses both energy demands and particular dietary requirements.

For effective weight monitoring and management, it is critical to prioritize nutrient-dense foods. Lean proteins, whole cereals, fruits, and vegetables are included. By distributing smaller, more frequent meals throughout the day, individuals with chronic bronchitis may find it easier to consume food, thereby alleviating the strain on the respiratory system during the process of digestion.

Engaging in regular physical activity is an essential element in maintaining optimal health and weight management for individuals diagnosed with chronic bronchitis.

It is imperative to seek guidance from healthcare professionals before commencing an exercise regimen. However, by incorporating moderate yoga, walking, or pulmonary rehabilitation exercises into one's routine, one can potentially enhance lung function and maintain a healthy weight.

Consistent weight monitoring is imperative, and any substantial fluctuations should be communicated to healthcare professionals. Substantial fluctuations in weight may serve as an indication of underlying concerns that necessitate medical attention.

Furthermore, healthcare experts are capable of offering recommendations regarding optimal caloric consumption, considering variables including age, gender, level of physical activity, and the extent of chronic bronchitis.

A Holistic Approach To Special Considerations For Chronic Bronchitis And Coexisting Conditions

Chronic bronchitis seldom occurs in isolation; coexisting conditions frequently necessitate particular attention in health management. Possible conditions that may be present include diabetes, cardiovascular ailments, or musculoskeletal disorders. Adopting a holistic approach to nutrition and healthcare is crucial for effectively addressing the unique challenges that chronic bronchitis and its comorbidities present.

When chronic bronchitis and cardiovascular disease are present, adherence to a heart-healthy diet is of therapeutic importance. This entails restricting the consumption of saturated and trans fats, decreasing sodium intake, and integrating foods that are abundant in fiber, potassium, and magnesium. Maintaining a balance between these dietary components can aid in the effective management of cardiovascular and respiratory health.

When chronic bronchitis and diabetes are present, it is critical to closely monitor carbohydrate consumption to regulate blood glucose levels. Optimizing portion sizes, dispersing carbohydrate consumption throughout the day, and selecting complex carbohydrates are all strategies that can aid in the management of diabetes and promote respiratory health.

Weight management efforts may be adversely affected by an individual's inability to participate in physical activity due to musculoskeletal issues. When this occurs, healthcare practitioners, such as physical therapists, can offer individualized exercise suggestions that account for limitations in mobility and promote general health.

It is imperative to adopt a collaborative approach that incorporates a multidisciplinary healthcare team to effectively manage the intricate dynamics that exist between chronic bronchitis and concurrent conditions. Consistent collaboration among specialists such as pulmonologists, dietitians, cardiologists, endocrinologists, and others guarantees the delivery of all-encompassing healthcare that attends to the unique requirements of each individual.

A Collaborative Journey With Healthcare Professionals And Dietitians

The effective management of chronic bronchitis via dietary interventions necessitates the cooperation of dietitians, healthcare professionals, and individuals. Precise guidance, education, and candid communication are fundamental elements of this collaborative endeavor.

Healthcare professionals have a critical responsibility in evaluating the extent of chronic bronchitis, detecting concurrent medical conditions, and formulating an all-encompassing course of treatment. Consistent medical examinations, pulmonary function assessments, and imaging investigations serve to monitor the disease's advancement and inform modifications to the treatment regimen.

Dietitians provide indispensable knowledge by customizing dietary regimens to address the specific requirements of patients afflicted with chronic bronchitis.

Dietitians are capable of developing individualized meal plans that target nutritional deficiencies, promote respiratory health, and conform to weight management objectives by conducting an extensive evaluation of dietary patterns, preferences, and medical background.

Education constitutes a foundational element of the collective endeavor. Chronic bronchitis patients would benefit from knowledge regarding the relationship between nutrition and their respiratory health as well as their overall well-being.

Healthcare professionals and dietitians possess the expertise to impart knowledge regarding the significance of regular physical activity, portion control, nutrient-dense food selection, and hydration.

Consistent consultations with healthcare practitioners and dietitians facilitate continuous modifications to the treatment regimen in response to individual progress and changing health requirements. By closely monitoring weight, nutritional status, and any observed symptomatic changes, one can adopt a proactive stance in the management of chronic bronchitis via nutritional means.

In summary, nutrition for individuals with chronic bronchitis extends beyond basic sustenance and is an essential element of comprehensive care that encompasses weight management, respiratory health, and concurrent medical conditions. Through the implementation of a balanced dietary regimen, vigilant weight monitoring, adherence to special dietary requirements, and effective collaboration with healthcare practitioners and dietitians, individuals afflicted with chronic bronchitis can augment their overall well-being and more efficiently navigate the complexities that accompany this persistent respiratory issue.

Conclusion

In conclusion, nutrition plays an indisputable role in the management of chronic bronchitis, providing a comprehensive strategy to enhance the well-being of those afflicted with this respiratory ailment. Patients with chronic bronchitis can benefit substantially from a well-balanced, nutrient-dense diet, which supports lung function, aids in the prevention of infections, and fortifies the immune system.

A diet rich in omega-3 fatty acids, fruits, and vegetables, which are known to have anti-inflammatory properties, could potentially mitigate the chronic inflammation that is linked to chronic bronchitis. Additionally, sufficient hydration is essential for sustaining optimal mucus production, which facilitates respiration and alleviates respiratory discomfort.

Additionally, those who have chronic bronchitis should exercise caution regarding potential food triggers that have the potential to worsen symptoms. Enhancing respiratory stability can be achieved by restricting the consumption of processed foods and avoiding irritants such as piquant foods and caffeine.

Customizing a nutrition plan to meet the specific requirements of individuals afflicted with chronic bronchitis ultimately requires the cooperation of healthcare professionals and those afflicted. Individuals afflicted with chronic bronchitis can improve their resilience, efficiently manage symptoms, and make strides toward a healthier and more active way of life by embracing a comprehensive approach to nutrition.

THE END

www.ingramcontent.com/pod-product-compliance
Lightning Source LLC
Chambersburg PA
CBHW060812260726
48660CB00002B/913